Copyright © 2023 by Monica Dimitrios

Table of Contents

LEUKEMIA

Leukemia is a broad term for cancers of the blood cells. The type of leukemia depends on the type of blood cell that becomes cancer and whether it grows quickly or slowly. Leukemia occurs most often in adults older than 55, but it is also the most common cancer in children younger than 15.

Prep Time: 40 mins

Total Time: 40 mins

Servings: 6

Ingredients

- 3 tablespoons extra-virgin olive oil, divided
- 1 pound 90% lean ground beef
- 2 teaspoons ground cumin
- ¾ teaspoon salt
- ¼ teaspoon ground pepper
- 3 medium Yukon Gold potatoes, diced (1/2-inch)
- 1 medium yellow onion, chopped
- 1 yellow bell pepper, diced (1/2-inch)
- 1 poblano pepper, diced (1/2-inch)
- 2 cloves garlic, minced
- 1 bunch lacinato kale, stemmed and roughly chopped
- 2 plum tomatoes, cored and diced (1/2-inch)
- 1 scallion, thinly sliced crosswise

Directions

1. Heat 1 tablespoon oil in a large cast-iron skillet over medium-high heat. Add beef, cumin, salt and pepper; cook, stirring often to break up the meat, until evenly browned, about 6 minutes. Using a slotted spoon, transfer the beef to a paper-towel-lined plate; do not wipe out the pan. Add 1 tablespoon oil to the drippings in the pan. Add potatoes; cook, stirring occasionally, until the potatoes begin to caramelize and are tender, about 20 minutes. Transfer the potatoes to the plate with the beef.

2. Heat the remaining 1 tablespoon oil in the skillet over medium heat. Add onion, bell pepper and poblano; cook, stirring occasionally, until tender, about 6 minutes. Add garlic; cook, stirring often, until aromatic, about 1 minute. Add kale and tomatoes; cook, stirring often, until the kale is wilted and the tomatoes are heated through, about 3 minutes. Stir in the beef and potatoes. Sprinkle with scallions, if desired.

2. One-Pot Garlicky Shrimp & Broccoli

Prep Time: 20 mins

Total Time: 20 mins

Servings: 4

Ingredients

- 3 tablespoons extra-virgin olive oil, divided
- 6 medium cloves garlic, sliced, divided
- 4 cups small broccoli florets
- ½ cup diced red bell pepper
- ½ teaspoon salt, divided
- ½ teaspoon ground pepper, divided
- 1 pound peeled and deveined raw shrimp (21-30 count)
- 2 teaspoons lemon juice, plus more to taste

Directions

1. Heat 2 tablespoons oil in a large saucepan over medium heat. Add half the garlic and cook until beginning to brown, about 1 minute. Add broccoli, bell pepper and 1/4 teaspoon each salt and pepper. Cover and cook, stirring once or twice and adding

1 tablespoon water if the pot is too dry, until the vegetables are tender, 3 to 5 minutes. Transfer to a bowl and keep warm.

2. Increase heat to medium-high and add the remaining 1 tablespoon oil to the pot. Add the remaining garlic and cook until beginning to brown, about 1 minute. Add shrimp and the remaining 1/4 teaspoon each salt and pepper; cook, stirring, until the shrimp are just cooked through, 3 to 5 minutes. Return the broccoli mixture to the pot along with lemon juice and stir to combine.

Total Time: 20 mins

Servings: 6

Ingredients

- 1 tablespoon extra-virgin olive oil
- 4 cups red cabbage, thinly sliced (about 1/4 large head)
- ¾ teaspoon caraway seeds
- ½ teaspoon salt
- 1 crisp, sweet apple, such as Braeburn or Gala, cut into matchsticks
- 1 shallot, minced
- 1 tablespoon red-wine vinegar
- ½ teaspoon Dijon mustard
- 1/2 teaspoon freshly, ground pepper
- 2 tablespoons chopped walnuts, toasted

Directions

1. Heat oil in a large saucepan over medium heat. Add cabbage, caraway seeds and salt. Cook, covered, stirring occasionally, until tender, 8 to 10 minutes. Remove from the heat. Add apple,

shallot, vinegar, mustard and pepper and stir until combined. Serve sprinkled with toasted walnuts.

4. Summer Skillet Vegetable & Egg Scramble

Prep Time: 30 mins

Total Time: 30 mins

Servings: 4

Ingredients

- 2 tablespoons olive oil
- 12 ounces baby potatoes, thinly sliced
- 4 cups thinly sliced vegetables, such as mushrooms, bell peppers, and/or zucchini (14 oz.)
- 3 scallions, thinly sliced, green and white parts separated
- 1 teaspoon minced fresh herbs, such as rosemary or thyme
- 6 large eggs (or 4 large eggs plus 4 egg whites), lightly beaten
- 2 cups packed leafy greens, such as baby spinach or baby kale
- ½ teaspoon salt

Directions

1. Heat oil in a large cast-iron or nonstick skillet over medium heat. Add potatoes; cover and cook, stirring several times, until they begin to soften, about 8 minutes.

2. Add sliced vegetables and scallion whites; cook uncovered, stirring occasionally, until the vegetables are tender and lightly browned, 8 to 10 minutes. Stir in herbs. Move the vegetable mixture to the perimeter of the pan.

3. Reduce heat to medium-low. Add eggs and scallion greens to the center of the pan. Cook, stirring, until the eggs are softly scrambled, about 2 minutes.

4. Stir leafy greens into the eggs. Remove from heat and stir to combine well. Stir in salt.

6. Spinach & Strawberry Meal-Prep Salad

Prep Time: 15 mins

Total Time: 30 mins

Servings: 4

Ingredients

- 1 pound boneless, skinless chicken thighs
- ½ teaspoon kosher salt
- ½ teaspoon dried thyme
- ½ teaspoon ground pepper
- 8 cups baby spinach
- 2 cups sliced strawberries
- ¼ cup feta cheese
- ¼ cup chopped toasted walnuts
- 6 tablespoons Balsamic Vinaigrette

Directions

1. Preheat oven to 400 degrees F. Line a baking sheet with parchment or foil.
2. Place chicken on the prepared baking sheet. Sprinkle all over with salt, thyme and pepper. Roast, flipping once, until the chicken is cooked

through and reaches an internal temperature of 165°F, 15 to 17 minutes. Set aside to cool, then slice into bite-size pieces.

3. Divide spinach among 4 single-serving lidded containers (2 cups each). Top each with one-fourth of the sliced chicken, 1/2 cup sliced strawberries, 1 tablespoon feta (if using) and 1 tablespoon walnuts.

4. Seal the salad containers and refrigerate for up to 4 days.

5. Transfer 1 1/2 tablespoons vinaigrette into each of 4 small lidded containers and refrigerate for up to 5 days.

6. Dress the salads with the vinaigrette just before serving.

Prep Time: 15 mins

Total Time: 15 mins

Servings: 4

Ingredients

- 8 ounces whole-wheat pasta
- 5 tablespoons extra-virgin olive oil
- 5 cloves garlic, chopped
- 1 teaspoon anchovy paste
- ¼ teaspoon crushed red pepper
- Zest and juice of 1 lemon
- 1 1/2 cups flaked cooked salmon
- 3 tablespoons chopped fresh parsley
- ¼ teaspoon salt
- 2 tablespoons whole-wheat breadcrumbs, toasted

Directions

1. Cook pasta according to package directions. Drain, reserving 1/2 cup cooking water.
2. Combine oil, garlic, anchovy paste, crushed red pepper, lemon zest and lemon juice in a large

skillet. Heat over medium-high heat until sizzling, about 3 minutes. Add the reserved water, the pasta, salmon, parsley and salt. Cook, stirring, until the sauce coats the pasta, about 2 minutes. Serve topped with breadcrumbs.

8. Grilled Salmon with Mustard & Herbs

Total Time: 40 mins

Servings: 4

Ingredients

- 2 lemons, thinly sliced, plus 1 lemon cut into wedges for garnish
- 20-30 sprigs mixed fresh herbs, plus 2 tablespoons chopped, divided
- 1 clove garlic
- ¼ teaspoon salt
- 1 tablespoon Dijon mustard
- 1 pound center-cut salmon, skinned

Directions

1. Preheat grill to medium-high.
2. Lay two 9-inch pieces of heavy-duty foil on top of each other and place on a rimless baking sheet. Arrange lemon slices in two layers in the center of the foil. Spread herb sprigs over the lemons. With the side of a chef's knife, mash garlic with salt to form a paste. Transfer to a small dish and stir in mustard and the remaining 2 tablespoons chopped

herbs. Spread the mixture over both sides of the salmon. Place the salmon on the herb sprigs.

3. Slide the foil and salmon off the baking sheet onto the grill without disturbing the salmon-lemon stack. Cover the grill; cook until the salmon is opaque in the center, 18 to 24 minutes. Wearing oven mitts, carefully transfer foil and salmon back onto the baking sheet. Cut the salmon into 4 portions and serve with lemon wedges (discard herb sprigs and lemon slices).

Total Time: 40 mins

Servings: 4

Ingredients

- 1 pound Brussels sprouts, trimmed and halved (or quartered if large)
- 4 small shallots, quartered
- 1 lemon, sliced
- 3 tablespoons extra-virgin olive oil, divided
- ¾ teaspoon salt, divided
- ½ teaspoon ground pepper, divided
- 2 cloves garlic, minced
- 1 tablespoon smoked paprika, sweet or hot
- 1 teaspoon dried thyme
- 4 large or 8 small bone-in chicken thighs (about 2 1/2 pounds), skin removed

Directions

1. Position rack in lower third of oven; preheat to 450 degrees F.

2. Combine Brussels sprouts, shallots and lemon with 2 tablespoons oil and 1/4 teaspoon each salt and pepper on a large rimmed baking sheet.

3. Mash garlic and the remaining 1/2 teaspoon salt with the side of a chef's knife to form a paste. Combine the garlic paste with paprika, thyme and the remaining 1 tablespoon oil and 1/4 teaspoon pepper in a small bowl. Rub the paste all over chicken. Nestle the chicken into the Brussels sprouts.

4. Roast on the lower rack until the Brussels sprouts are tender and an instant-read thermometer inserted into the thickest part of the chicken without touching bone registers 165 degrees F, 20 to 25 minutes.

10. Oven-Roasted Squash with Garlic & Parsley

Total Time: 1 hr

Servings: 10

Ingredients

- 5 pounds winter squash (such as butternut, buttercup, kabocha or hubbard), peeled, seeded and cut into 1-inch chunks
- 2 tablespoons extra-virgin olive oil, divided
- 1 ½ teaspoons salt
- ¼ teaspoon freshly ground pepper, divided
- 3 cloves garlic, minced
- 2 tablespoons chopped Italian parsley

Directions

1. Preheat oven to 375 degrees F.
2. Toss squash with 4 teaspoons oil, salt and 1/4 teaspoon pepper. Spread evenly on a large baking sheet. Roast, stirring occasionally, until tender throughout and lightly browned, 30 to 45 minutes (depending on the variety of squash).
3. Heat the remaining 2 teaspoons oil in a small skillet over medium heat. Add garlic and cook,

stirring, until fragrant but not brown, 30 seconds to 1 minute. Toss the roasted squash with the garlic and parsley. Taste, adjust the seasoning and serve.

Total Time: 45 mins

Servings: 4

Ingredients

- 2 tablespoons whole-grain or Dijon mustard
- 2 tablespoons chopped fresh thyme or 2 teaspoons dried
- 2 tablespoons extra-virgin olive oil, divided
- ½ teaspoon salt, divided
- ½ teaspoon freshly ground pepper, divided
- 1 1/2-2 pounds bone-in chicken thighs, skin removed
- 2 medium sweet potatoes, peeled and cut into 1-inch pieces
- 1 large red onion, cut into 1-inch wedges

Directions

1. Position rack in lower third of oven; preheat to 450 degrees F. Place a large rimmed baking sheet in the oven to preheat.

2. Combine mustard, thyme, 1 tablespoon oil and 1/4 teaspoon each salt and pepper in a small bowl; spread the mixture evenly on chicken.

3. Toss sweet potatoes and onion in a bowl with the remaining 1 tablespoon oil and 1/4 teaspoon each salt and pepper. Carefully remove the baking sheet from the oven and spread the vegetables on it. Place the chicken on top of the vegetables.

4. Return the pan to the oven and roast, stirring the vegetables once halfway through, until the vegetables are tender and beginning to brown and an instant-read thermometer inserted into a chicken thigh registers 165 degrees F, 30 to 35 minutes.

Prep Time: 35 mins

Total Time: 35 mins

Servings: 4

Ingredients

- 2 bell peppers, any color
- 1 avocado, diced
- ½ cup diced red onion
- 1 jalapeño pepper, minced
- ½ cup chopped fresh cilantro, plus more for garnish
- 2 tomatoes, seeded and diced
- Juice of 1 lime
- ¾ teaspoon salt, divided
- 2 teaspoons olive oil, divided
- 8 large eggs
- ¼ teaspoon ground pepper, divided

Directions

1. Slice tops and bottoms off bell peppers and finely dice. Remove and discard seeds and membranes. Slice each pepper into four 1/2-inch-thick rings.
2. Combine the diced pepper with avocado, onion, jalapeño, cilantro, tomatoes, lime juice, and 1/2 teaspoon salt in a medium bowl.

3. Heat 1 teaspoon oil in a large nonstick skillet over medium heat. Add 4 bell pepper rings, then crack 1 egg into the middle of each ring. Season with 1/8 teaspoon each salt and pepper. Cook until the whites are mostly set but the yolks are still runny, 2 to 3 minutes. Gently flip and cook 1 minute more for runny yolks, 1 1/2 to 2 minutes more for firmer yolks. Transfer to serving plates and repeat with the remaining pepper rings and eggs.
4. Serve with the avocado salsa and garnish with additional cilantro, if desired.

Prep Time: 15 mins

Total Time: 1 hr

Servings: 4

Ingredients

- 1 pound Yukon Gold or red potatoes, cubed
- 1 pound mushrooms (shiitake, cremini, oyster or other fresh mushrooms), trimmed and sliced
- 2 tablespoons extra-virgin olive oil, divided
- ¼ teaspoon salt
- ¼ teaspoon ground pepper
- 2 cloves garlic, peeled and sliced
- 14 ounces halibut, grouper or cod fillet, cut into 4 portions
- 4 tablespoons lemon juice
- 1 teaspoon herbes de Provence
- Fresh thyme for garnish

Directions

1. Preheat oven to 425 degrees F.

2. Toss potatoes, mushrooms, 1 Tbsp. oil, salt, and pepper in a large bowl. Transfer to a 9x13-inch baking dish. Roast until the vegetables are just tender, 30 to 40 minutes.

3. Stir the vegetables, then stir in garlic. Place fish on top. Drizzle with lemon juice and the remaining 1 Tbsp. oil. Sprinkle with herbes de Provence. Bake until the fish is opaque in the center and flakes easily, 10 to 15 minutes. Garnish with thyme, if desired.

14. Greek Salad Dressing

Prep Time: 5 mins

Total Time 5 mins

Servings: 7

Ingredients

- 3 tablespoons extra-virgin olive oil
- 1 tablespoon lemon juice
- 1 tablespoon red-wine vinegar
- 1 teaspoon dried oregano
- ¼ teaspoon salt
- ¼ teaspoon ground pepper

Directions

1. Whisk oil, lemon juice, vinegar, oregano, salt and pepper in a small bowl or shake in a small jar. Use immediately or refrigerate for up to 1 week.

15. Herb-Roasted Turkey

Prep Time: 30 mins

Total Time 3 hrs 30 mins

Servings: 12

Ingredients

- 1 10- to 12-pound turkey
- ¼ cup fresh herbs, plus 20 whole sprigs, such as thyme, rosemary, sage, oregano and/or marjoram, divided
- 2 tablespoons canola oil
- 1 teaspoon salt
- 1 teaspoon freshly ground pepper
- Aromatics, onion, apple, lemon and/or orange, cut into 2-inch pieces (1 1/2 cups)
- 3 cups water, plus more as needed

Directions

1. Position a rack in the lower third of the oven; preheat to 475 degrees F.
2. Remove giblets and neck from turkey cavities and reserve for making gravy. Place the turkey, breast-

side up, on a rack in a large roasting pan; pat dry with paper towels. Mix minced herbs, oil, salt and pepper in a small bowl. Rub the herb mixture all over the turkey, under the skin and onto the breast meat. Place aromatics and 10 of the herb sprigs in the cavity. Tuck the wing tips under the turkey. Tie the legs together with kitchen string. Add 3 cups water and the remaining 10 herb sprigs to the pan.

3. Roast the turkey until the skin is golden brown, 45 minutes. Remove from the oven. Cover the breast with a double layer of foil, cutting as necessary to conform to the breast.

4. Reduce oven temperature to 350° and continue roasting until an instant-read thermometer inserted into the thickest part of a thigh without touching bone registers 165°, 1 1/4 to 1 3/4 hours more. If the pan dries out, tilt the turkey to let juices run out of the cavity and into the pan and add 1 cup water.

5. Transfer the turkey to a serving platter and cover with foil. Let the turkey rest for 20 minutes. Remove string and carve.

Prep Time: 30 mins

Total Time: 30 mins

Servings: 4

Ingredients

- ¼ cup 1/2-inch pieces sweet potato
- ¼ cup 1/2-inch pieces yellow sweet pepper
- ¼ cup coarsely chopped fresh broccoli
- 8 omega-3 enriched eggs
- 1 teaspoon snipped fresh basil
- ½ teaspoon snipped fresh thyme
- ⅛ teaspoon salt
- ⅛ teaspoon cracked black pepper
- 1 avocado, halved, seeded, peeled and thinly sliced
- 5 ½ cups grape or cherry tomatoes, halved
- Sriracha sauce

Directions

1. Preheat oven to 350 F. Coat an oven-going 10-inch nonstick skillet with cooking spray. Add sweet

potato, sweet pepper and broccoli; cook and stir over medium 5 to 7 minutes or until tender.

2. In a medium bowl whisk together eggs, basil, thyme, salt and black pepper. Pour mixture over vegetables in skillet. Cook, without stirring, until mixture begins to set on bottom and around edges. Using a spatula, lift egg mixture so uncooked portion flows underneath.

3. Transfer skillet to oven; cook 5 minutes or until egg mixture is set. Remove from oven. Let stand 2 minutes. Top servings with avocado and tomatoes. Drizzle with sriracha.

17. Cucumber & Avocado Salad

Prep Time: 5 mins

Total Time: 20 mins

Servings: 4

Ingredients

- 1 medium shallot, thinly sliced crosswise and separated into rings
- 3 tablespoons fresh lime juice
- 3 tablespoons extra-virgin olive oil
- 1 tablespoon thinly sliced fresh mint
- 1 tablespoon thinly sliced fresh basil
- ½ teaspoon salt
- 1 English cucumber, thinly sliced
- 1 ripe avocado, halved, pitted and sliced crosswise

Directions

1. Toss shallot rings with lime juice in a large bowl; let stand until softened, about 10 minutes. Whisk in oil, mint, basil and salt. Add cucumber; toss to coat. Let the cucumber marinate in the dressing,

tossing occasionally, until softened, about 10 minutes.

2. Using a slotted spoon, transfer the cucumber to a platter; top with avocado. Drizzle the dressing over the salad. Serve immediately.

Prep Time: 10 mins

Total Time: 25 mins

Servings: 2

Ingredients

- Cooking spray
- 2 (7.5 ounce) cans unsalted pink salmon (with skin and bones)
- 1 large egg
- ½ cup whole-wheat panko breadcrumbs
- 2 tablespoons chopped fresh dill
- 2 tablespoons canola mayonnaise
- 2 teaspoons Dijon mustard
- ¼ teaspoon ground pepper
- 2 lemon wedges

Directions

1. Coat the basket of an air fryer with cooking spray.
2. Drain salmon; remove and discard any large bones and skin. Place the salmon in a medium bowl. Add egg, panko, dill, mayonnaise, mustard and pepper;

stir gently until combined. Shape the mixture into four 3-inch-diameter cakes.

3. Coat the cakes with cooking spray; place in the prepared basket. Cook at 400 degrees F until browned and an instant-read thermometer inserted into the thickest portion registers 160 degrees F, about 12 minutes. Serve with lemon wedges.

Prep Time: 10 mins

Total Time: 3 hrs 45 mins

Servings: 8

Ingredients

- 1 medium butternut squash (2-2 1/2 pounds), peeled, seeded and cubed (about 5 cups)
- 3 cups "no-chicken" broth or vegetable broth
- 1 medium onion, chopped
- 4 teaspoons curry powder
- ½ teaspoon garlic powder
- ¾ teaspoon salt
- 1 (14 ounce) can coconut milk
- 1-2 tablespoons lime juice, plus wedges for serving
- Chopped fresh cilantro for garnish

Directions

1. Stir squash, broth, onion, curry powder, garlic powder and salt together in a 5-quart slow cooker. Cover and cook until the vegetables are very tender, 7 hours on Low or 3 1/2 hours on High.

Turn off heat and stir in coconut milk and lime juice to taste. Puree with an immersion blender until smooth. Garnish with cilantro.

20. Roasted Butternut Squash Seeds

Prep Time: 5 mins

Total Time: 30 mins

Servings: 2

Ingredients

- ¼ cup butternut squash seeds, rinsed and patted dry
- ½ teaspoon extra-virgin olive oil
- Pinch of salt

Directions

1. Preheat oven to 325°F. Toss squash seeds, oil and salt together on a large rimmed baking sheet; spread in a single layer. Roast, stirring halfway through, until the seeds start to pop and are lightly browned, 14 to 15 minutes. Let cool on the baking sheet for 10 minutes.

21. Lemon-Blueberry Nice Cream

Prep Time: 10 mins

Total Time: 10 mins

Servings: 4

Ingredients

- 3 medium ripe bananas, sliced and frozen
- ¼ cup lemon juice
- ¼ teaspoon vanilla extract
- ¼ cup cold water, as needed
- ¾ cup frozen blueberries

Directions

1. Place frozen banana slices, lemon juice and vanilla in a food processor. Process until smooth, adding cold water to loosen the mixture, if necessary. Transfer to a bowl; stir in frozen blueberries. Serve immediately or store in an airtight container in the freezer for up to 1 month.

22. Miso-Maple Salmon

Prep Time: 15 mins

Total Time: 15 mins

Servings: 8

Ingredients

- 2 lemons
- 2 limes
- ¼ cup white miso
- 2 tablespoons extra-virgin olive oil
- 2 tablespoons maple syrup
- ¼ teaspoon ground pepper
- Pinch of cayenne pepper
- 1 (2 1/2 pound) skin-on salmon fillet
- Sliced scallions for garnish

Directions

1. Position rack in upper third of oven; preheat broiler to high. Line a large rimmed baking sheet with foil.
2. Juice 1 lemon and 1 lime into a small bowl. Whisk in miso, oil, maple syrup, pepper and cayenne.

Place salmon, skin-side down, on the prepared pan and spread the miso mixture on top. Halve the remaining lemon and lime and arrange around the salmon, cut-sides up.

3. Broil the salmon just until it flakes with a fork, 7 to 12 minutes. Serve with the lemon and lime halves and sprinkle with scallions, if desired.

Prep Time: 5 mins

Total Time: 25 mins

Servings: 4

Ingredients

- 1 medium butternut squash, cubed (3/4-inch; about 4 cups)
- 2 teaspoons extra-virgin olive oil
- ½ teaspoon ground paprika
- ¼ teaspoon salt
- ¼ teaspoon ground pepper
- ⅛ teaspoon garlic powder

Directions

1. Preheat air fryer to 400°F for 3 minutes. Meanwhile, toss squash, oil, paprika, salt, pepper and garlic powder together in a large bowl.
2. Lightly coat the fry basket with cooking spray. Add the prepared squash to the basket; cook for 10 minutes. After 10 minutes, open the fryer and lightly toss the squash to redistribute; cook until

lightly browned and crispy on edges, about 10 minutes more.

24. Almond Butter & Banana Protein Smoothie

Total Time: 5 mins

Servings: 1

Ingredients

- 1 small frozen banana
- 1 cup unsweetened almond milk
- 2 tablespoons almond butter
- 2 tablespoons unflavored protein powder
- 1 tablespoon sweetener of your choice
- ½ teaspoon ground cinnamon
- 4-6 ice cubes

Directions

1. Combine all ingredients in a blender and blend until smooth.

Prep Time: 45 mins

Total Time: 45 mins

Servings: 4

Ingredients

- 3 tablespoons extra-virgin olive oil, divided
- 8 ounces Italian sausage (about 3 links), casing removed
- 1 cup diced onion
- ½ cup diced carrot
- ½ cup diced celery
- 2 tablespoons finely chopped garlic
- 2 teaspoons paprika, preferably smoked
- 12 ounces baby yellow potatoes, sliced
- 8 ounces Brussels sprouts, trimmed and sliced
- 4 cups low-sodium chicken broth
- 2 tablespoons red-wine vinegar
- ½ teaspoon salt
- ½ teaspoon ground pepper
- ¼ cup chopped flat-leaf parsley

Directions

1. Heat 1 tablespoon oil in a large pot over medium heat. Add sausage and cook, stirring occasionally and breaking up with the spoon, until browned, 4 to 6 minutes. Transfer to a plate.

2. Add the remaining 2 tablespoons oil, onion, carrot and celery to the pot; cook, stirring occasionally, until softened, about 5 minutes. Add garlic and paprika; cook, stirring, for 30 seconds. Add potatoes, Brussels sprouts and broth; bring to a boil over high heat. Reduce heat to a simmer and cook, stirring occasionally, until the potatoes are tender, 6 to 8 minutes.

3. Stir in the sausage, vinegar, salt and pepper. Serve sprinkled with parsley.

26. One-Pot Vegetable Soup with Cabbage

Prep Time: 35 mins

Total Time: 35 mins

Servings: 8

Ingredients

- 2 tablespoons extra-virgin olive oil
- 1 10-ounce bag frozen seasoning blend, thawed
- 3 cloves garlic, thinly sliced
- 1 ½ teaspoons smoked paprika
- 4 cups lower-sodium vegetable broth
- 2 cups water
- 1 (14.5 ounce) can fire-roasted diced tomatoes, undrained
- 1 medium head green cabbage, cored and chopped
- 3 small Yukon Gold potatoes, peeled and chopped
- 2 tablespoons chopped fresh thyme, plus more for garnish
- ¾ teaspoon salt
- 2 tablespoons plus 2 teaspoons lemon juice
- Lemon wedges for serving

Directions

1. Heat oil in a large Dutch oven or other large heavy pot over medium-high heat. Add seasoning blend; cook, stirring occasionally, until tender, about 5 minutes. Add garlic and paprika; cook, stirring constantly, until fragrant, about 30 seconds. Stir in broth, water, tomatoes, cabbage, potatoes, thyme and salt; bring to a boil over high heat. Reduce heat to medium-low; cover and simmer, stirring occasionally, until the cabbage and potatoes are tender, about 25 minutes. Remove from heat and divide among 8 bowls; stir in 1 teaspoon lemon juice per bowl. Garnish with additional thyme, if desired, and serve with lemon wedges.

27. Skillet Lemon-Pepper Salmon

Prep Time: 15 mins

Total Time: 15 mins

Servings: 4

Ingredients

- 4 (5-6 oz) skin-on salmon fillets, preferably wild Alaskan
- 1 teaspoon cracked black pepper
- ½ teaspoon paprika
- ½ teaspoon garlic powder
- ½ teaspoon salt
- 1 teaspoon grated lemon zest
- 2 tablespoons lemon juice, divided
- 1 tablespoon extra-virgin olive oil
- 2 tablespoons finely chopped fresh parsley
- Pinch of flaky sea salt

Directions

1. Pat salmon dry and place, skin-side down, in a medium bowl. Sprinkle with pepper, paprika,

garlic powder, 1/2 teaspoon salt and 1 tablespoon lemon juice.

2. Heat oil in a large nonstick pan over medium-high heat until shimmering. Add the salmon, skin-side down; cook until the skin releases from the pan easily and the edges are opaque, about 4 minutes. Reduce heat to low and flip the salmon. Continue cooking until an instant-read thermometer inserted in the thickest part of the salmon registers 145°F, 3 to 5 minutes .

3. Sprinkle the salmon with the remaining 1 tablespoon lemon juice, lemon zest, parsley and flaky salt.

28. Steamed Butternut Squash

Prep Time: 15 mins

Total Time: 30 mins

Servings: 10

Ingredients

- 1 (20 ounce) package cubed peeled butternut squash
- Local Offers

Directions

1. Bring 1 inch of water to boil in a large saucepan fitted with a steamer basket.
2. Add squash. Cover and steam until very tender, about 15 minutes.

29. Lemon-Garlic Vegetable Soup

Prep Time: 20 mins

Total Time: 40 mins

Servings: 4

Ingredients

- 2 tablespoons extra-virgin olive oil
- 1 small onion, chopped
- 4 large cloves garlic, minced
- 2 cups halved green beans
- 1 medium zucchini, diced
- 2 ears corn, kernels cut from the cob
- 4 cups low-sodium vegetable broth
- 3 cups chopped stemmed kale
- 2 medium tomatoes, diced
- ½ teaspoon salt
- ¼ teaspoon ground pepper
- 4 teaspoons lemon juice, plus more to taste
- ¼ cup chopped fresh herbs, such as basil, cilantro, tarragon or parsley

Directions

1. Heat oil in a large pot over medium heat. Add onion; cook, stirring, until starting to soften, about 2 minutes. Add garlic; cook, stirring, until fragrant, about 30 seconds. Add green beans, zucchini and corn; cook, stirring, for 2 minutes. Add broth, kale, tomatoes, salt and pepper; increase heat to high and bring to a boil. Reduce heat to maintain a simmer; cook until the vegetables are soft, 12 to 15 minutes. Remove from heat and stir in lemon juice and herbs.

Prep Time: 25 mins

Total Time: 25 mins

Servings: 4

Ingredients

- ⅓ cup prepared pesto
- 2 tablespoons balsamic vinegar
- 1 tablespoon extra-virgin olive oil
- ½ teaspoon salt
- ¼ teaspoon ground pepper
- 1 pound peeled and deveined large shrimp (16-20 count), patted dry
- 4 cups arugula
- 2 cups cooked quinoa
- 1 cup halved cherry tomatoes
- 1 avocado, diced

Directions

1. Whisk pesto, vinegar, oil, salt and pepper in a large bowl. Remove 4 tablespoons of the mixture to a small bowl; set both bowls aside.

2. Heat a large cast-iron skillet over medium-high heat. Add shrimp and cook, stirring, until just cooked through with a slight char, 4 to 5 minutes. Remove to a plate.

3. Add arugula and quinoa to the large bowl with the vinaigrette and toss to coat. Divide the arugula mixture between 4 bowls. Top with tomatoes, avocado and shrimp. Drizzle each bowl with 1 tablespoon of the reserved pesto mixture.

Prep Time: 45 mins

Total Time: 1 hr 30 mins

Servings: 6

Ingredients

- 1 ¼ cups water
- 3 tablespoons tomato paste
- 2 tablespoons rice vinegar
- 2 tablespoons reduced-sodium soy sauce
- 4 tablespoons hoisin sauce, divided
- 2 tablespoons minced fresh ginger, divided
- 4 cloves garlic, minced, divided
- ½ teaspoon crushed red pepper
- 2 tablespoons cornstarch
- 12 large leaves savoy cabbage
- 2 cups finely chopped broccoli
- 1 pound lean ground pork
- 1 ½ cups cooked brown rice
- 1 bunch scallions, sliced
- 1 teaspoon toasted sesame oil

Directions

Preheat oven to 400°F. Coat a 9-by-13-inch baking dish with cooking spray.

Whisk water, tomato paste, vinegar, soy sauce, 2 tablespoons hoisin, 1 tablespoon ginger, 2 cloves garlic and crushed red pepper in a small saucepan. Whisk in cornstarch; bring to a simmer over medium-high heat. Cook, stirring, until thickened, about 2 minutes. Remove from heat and set aside.

Meanwhile, bring a large pot of water to a boil. Add 4 cabbage leaves and cook, gently stirring, until softened, 1 to 2 minutes. Transfer to a rimmed baking sheet. Repeat with the remaining cabbage leaves. Place broccoli in a colander and pour the hot water over it. Refresh with cold water. Transfer to a large bowl. Add pork, rice, scallions, sesame oil, the remaining 2 tablespoons hoisin, 1 tablespoon ginger and 2 cloves garlic, and 3 tablespoons of the reserved sauce. Stir to combine well.

Place 1/3 cup filling over the bottom third of 1 softened cabbage leaf. Fold the bottom and sides over the filling and roll up. Place, seam-side down, in the prepared baking dish. Repeat with the remaining leaves and filling. Pour the remaining sauce over the rolls. Cover with foil and bake until an instant-read thermometer inserted into the center of a roll registers 150°F, about 40 minutes.